M000281854

BONDAGE

Lord Morpheous

QUIVER

Brimming with creative inspiration, how-to projects, and useful
information to enrich your everyday life, Quarto Knows is a favorite
destination for those pursuing their interests and passions. Visit our
site and dig deeper with our books into your area of interest:
Quarto Creates, Quarto Cooks, Quarto Homes, Quarto Lives,
Quarto Drives, Quarto Explores, Quarto Gifts, or Quarto Kids.

© 2017 Quarto Publishing Group USA Inc.

First Published in 2017 by Fair Winds Press, an imprint of The Quarto Group,
100 Cummings Center, Suite 265-D, Beverly, MA 01915, USA.
T (978) 282-9590 F (978) 283-2742 QuartoKnows.com

All rights reserved. No part of this book may be reproduced in any form without written
permission of the copyright owners. All images in this book have been reproduced
with the knowledge and prior consent of the artists concerned, and no responsibility
is accepted by producer, publisher, or printer for any infringement of copyright or
otherwise, arising from the contents of this publication. Every effort has been made to
ensure that credits accurately comply with information supplied. We apologize for any
inaccuracies that may have occurred and will resolve inaccurate or missing information in
a subsequent reprinting of the book.

Fair Winds Press titles are also available at discount for retail, wholesale, promotional,
and bulk purchase. For details, contact the Special Sales Manager by email at
specialsales@quarto.com or by mail at The Quarto Group, Attn: Special Sales Manager,
401 Second Avenue North, Suite 310, Minneapolis, MN 55401, USA.

The Publisher maintains the records relating to images in this book required by 18 USC
2257. Records are located at The Quarto Group, 100 Cummings Center, Suite 265-D,
Beverly, MA 01915, USA.

The content for this book originally appeared in *Bondage Basics* (Quiver Books, 2015) by
Lord Morpheous.

21 20 19   3 4 5

ISBN: 978-1-59233-793-4

Digital edition published in 2017

Library of Congress Cataloging-in-Publication Data available

Cover design/illustration: www.gordonbeveridge.com
Book design by Sporto
Photography by Holly Randall, Lord Morpheous, and Geoff George Photography

Printed and bound in Hong Kong

Contents

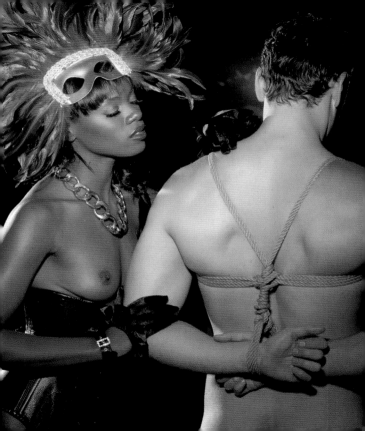

ALL ABOUT KINK

Regardless of what they'd like you to believe, absolutely everyone has a kink.

An individual's kink may even seem at odds with how that person is in "real life." This is because our kinks offer us an escape from stress; they create a space in which we can truly be ourselves, outside of all the expectations of those around us. They let us express ourselves emotionally, artistically, sexually—in any way that you can think of. They give us confidence and allow us to grow. This is one of the reasons why I wrote this book—to shed light on rope bondage art as a sensual medium and help people create their own art (and hopefully be sexually titillated all the while).

When we first begin to explore the kinky sides of our sexual personalities, it can feel scary, as if we're catapulting ourselves into a world that we don't understand. The aim of this book is not to tell you what you should like, but to help you explore your sexuality and artistic abilities and to imbue you with rope bondage skills.

This book is inspired by the work of many rope and bondage artists. Lew Rubens' work made practicing rope techniques much easier, especially with the approach Lew took, inspired by long-ago Western bondage masters such as John Willie. I learned the beauty of making bondage simple and utilitarian, leaving room for inspiration and flourishes.

Another great friend, Midori, gave me hands-on training in Japanese-style bondage. She always said that the work could never be "truly Japanese," because there were differences in the way she tied and what was taking place in Japan. Nevertheless, it was great instruction in Eastern knot tying.

I became inspired by Arisue Go and Osada Steve and the work I saw in Japanese books. However, I never strayed far from my Western roots and incorporated as much of my own style into what I was seeing and practicing. One of the most satisfying aspects was to work out problems with knots in my own style with the skills I had developed.

That passion is what drove me to create and host the world's largest public rope bondage event called Morpheous' Bondage Extravaganza (MBE). The event takes place in Toronto annually in October. It showcases the best rope bondage artists around the world. The event now takes place concurrently in different cities around the world.

We all come to rope bondage in different ways, and our paths through it will be equally different. Perhaps you've felt the soft tug of rope against your fleshy bits while playing with a partner. Perhaps you viewed a rope bondage exhibition once and felt a stirring in a place that you've never felt before. Perhaps you saw this book in a store and picked it up on impulse. No matter how you arrived here, I hope that this book will be the first step on a journey that takes you wherever you want to go—and beyond where you think you might end up, all while having fun and playing safely.

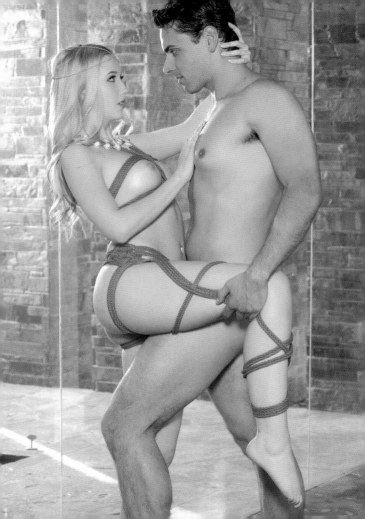

Chapter 1

BONDAGE 101

If you've picked up this book, I'm going to assume that you're interested in bringing a little more kink into your life. Welcome to the filthy, exciting world of bondage.

But first, the basics: Bondage is the practice of tying or restraining a partner for sexual or artistic purposes. In this book, we'll be talking mostly about bondage with rope, simply because it is the most fun. Bondage is often discussed in the wider category of BDSM, as it tends to overlap with other kinky activities. Your journey through rope bondage is your own, and you should find your own path.

Let's start from the very beginning. What does BDSM mean?

BDSM describes three concepts of bondage and discipline, dominance and submission, and sadism and masochism. Sadism is the experience of pleasure through inflicting pain, while masochism is the experience of pleasure while receiving pain. This also describes the fluid sexuality that can allow people to enjoy being both dominant and submissive, or both giving and receiving pleasure through pain.

BDSM relationships in popular culture have left a lot of people thinking that these relationhips must be abusive. This is far from the truth. The BDSM community values trust, safety, and communication above all else and engages in pain for pleasure only in a consensual setting. Even if BDSM is a new concept to you, you've probably strayed closer to BDSM-style sexual expression than you think—for example, if you've experienced a little pain for pleasure. If not, don't worry. That's what this book is for.

BDSM activities range in intensity, and almost anything, when done right, can come under the BDSM umbrella. Tying your husband's wrists to the bedframe with his neckties and making him watch you do a striptease is BDSM; so is buying your first 6-inch (15 cm) strap-on and making him beg you to use it on him. There are a million and one different ways to enjoy BDSM and you should never feel pressured to go beyond your own personal boundaries—although exploring where exactly your boundaries lie is part of the fun!

In this book, however, we're going to focus on the bondage and discipline part of BDSM, and more specifically on the bondage element. This includes bondage using rope and household items such as scarves, belts, and men's ties. I will show you how to make it safe and sexy at the same time.

FINDING YOUR ROLE

When you're first beginning to explore your kinky side, it can be difficult to know just what type of role will fit you best. You might love to tie your partner's arms and legs to the bed to play with him or her, but are you ready for the responsibility of someone else giving himself or herself up to you totally?

It's important to remember that there are a multitude of roles in BDSM and that the whole spectrum of human sexuality can never be boiled down to just one or two narrow categories. That said, some people find great comfort in moving from one role to another, as the boundaries therein can help them explore all possible experiences. No one can ever tell you which role is right for you; rather, the way to find your role is to experiment, keep an open mind, and try each one on.

You might still have questions after your first or many play sessions. That's okay; some people never feel comfortable putting labels on themselves and instead prefer to exist in the fluid, fluctuating space of sexuality that BDSM easily allows. BDSM is a journey, and if you never quite find a destination, you're still in for a hell of a lot of fun.

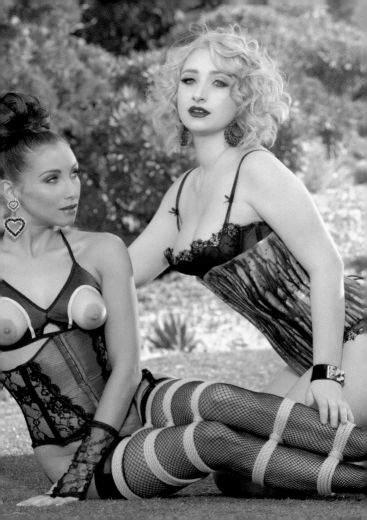

AFTERCARE

They say that what goes up must come down, and this is just as true for BDSM. During play, the submissives in a scene sometimes reach a state known as subspace, in which all cares, troubles, and pain fall away and the sub exists in a dream state of euphoria. It can feel similar to being drunk or high on drugs, and the feelings after this sensation subsides can also be the same as those coming off drugs.

The phenomenon of coming down after a scene is known as subdrop. This is caused by endorphins leaving your body and sending you into withdrawal. The intensity of this "down" feeling can range from a few hours of feeling sad, vulnerable, or physically exhausted to a week of feeling numb and a little lost. It's important that everyone leaves a scene feeling cared for and nurtured; any play session, even light bondage, requires aftercare. You should also discuss aftercare in your negotiation process with any new partner. The negotiation process is the period before play begins, in which you lay down all ground rules and boundaries, talk about any health issues that may affect play, and ensure that all parties are comfortable. Aftercare is as necessary as foreplay in the BDSM world—and can be just as erotic.

◀ *Are you ready for someone to give him- or herself up to you totally?*

The physical effects of a scene, such as any cuts, bruises, and abrasions, should be sterilized and bandaged. Apply arnica to help heal bruising, and drink plenty of water. Seek immediate medical attention immediately for any serious injury.

Emotional aftercare can take many forms, but the dominant in the scene should ensure that the space is comforting and should also address any feelings that the sub expresses, as well as providing positive reinforcement, which can be as simple as "you're a good little thing, yes, you are." Soft physical contact can be reassuring for some people, and good-quality dark chocolate can help with subdrop.

Sometimes it's necessary to provide yourself with aftercare, if your play partners aren't available after the scene or you prefer to be alone. It's good to have a little "aftercare pack" for yourself, so you can make yourself comfortable and deal with feelings that may arise. It might include a letter from a lover, body cream, your favorite movie, relaxing music, candles, incense, or candies. Call someone if you're feeling lonely.

ROPE BONDAGE AND BDSM

Bondage in BDSM refers to the practice of tying up or restraining a partner (or "rope bunny") for sexual activity, decoration, power play, or art. Not all rope bondage is for sexual play. In fact, rope as an art form has a long history. My annual rope bondage display, Morpheous' Bondage

Extravaganza, showcases the beauty of rope art, and its huge attendance proves that rope art can be gorgeous even to those outside the scene. Some people may not enjoy being hogtied and flogged; instead they might enjoy toe cuffs or having their fingers, hands, feet, or bodies tied up with colored wool. There are many functions of bondage that are neither sexual nor artistic. For instance, finger or toe bondage can keep your service-oriented slave in the correct mind-set to serve you, and a crude rope chastity belt can remind your submissive who she belongs to while she's at work. Some bunnies love the feel of rough jute rope against their skin while they're teased and tickled; others enjoy the headspace that bondage puts them into, without needing any extra stimulation. There is no right way to incorporate bondage into your life, and finding out what floats your boat is half the fun!

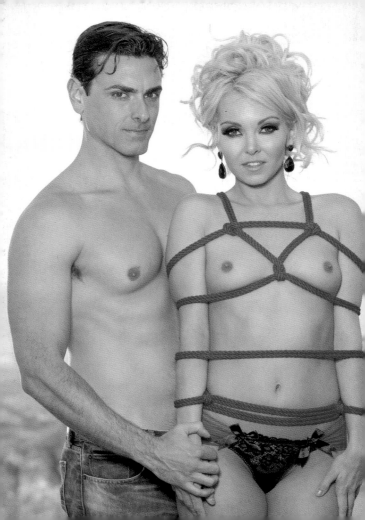

Chapter 2

COMMUNICATION AND SAFETY

George Bernard Shaw said, "The single biggest problem in communication is the illusion that it has taken place." Now the Irish playwright wasn't exactly known to be a player in Dublin's turn-of-the-century kink scene, but he still perfectly understood the central danger that exists in rope bondage play: bad communication.

In rope bondage, if all participants don't know the rules, then injuries sustained can be mental as well as physical. This goes for any play where there's an exchange of power and one party is given total responsibility for the pleasure and well-being of another.

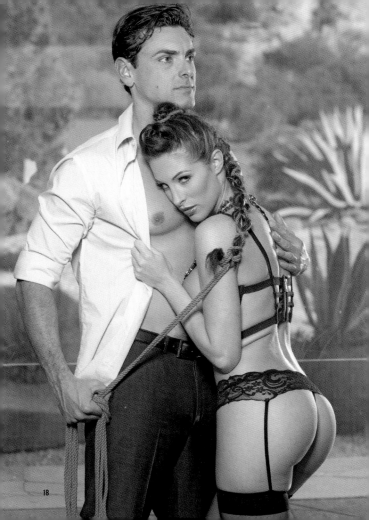

COMMUNICATION, COMMUNICATION, COMMUNICATION

It's something of a cliché, but it's true: Communication is the key to safe, sexy, and fulfilling play. Safe sex is sexy sex. It begins long before the rope is uncoiled and it's still going on when your heartbeats finally return to a resting state.

Whether you're taking your first steps into bondage with a partner or partners, going hand-in-hand with someone who's more experienced, or even if you're a single looking to find someone to explore with, your first conversation with any potential partner should be open, honest, and thorough. You should talk about your desires, turn-ons, and fantasies, but you also need to talk about your boundaries, turn-offs, and concerns. Tell your partner if you're claustrophobic, if you don't like having your wrists bound together, or if you have any medical conditions, like an old shoulder injury. Be clear and honest with them especially if you have experienced mental or physical abuse in the past. Your partner should also share this information with you, and remember: Though you may not see its significance, your partner will. Always listen and be empathetic. Empathy is key, and if you feel your partner doesn't value it or has a problem with it, then look for another partner.

◄ *Communication is key to any relationship—but it's even more important in rope bondage.*

Once you've shared your issues, now comes the fun part: Laying down your deepest, darkest fantasies. Share your dirtiest dreams and listen to your partner's. It's the most fun you can have with your clothes on!

When you're finally comfortable with your partner, and you're confident that he or she knows and understands your mindset, start setting boundaries or ground rules. Every person has hard and soft limits. Hard limits are lines that you simply will not cross and don't even want to approach. Your hard limit might be golden showers, or forced lesbianism, or even having your eyes covered; no one will judge your limits, and if they do, find a new partner. Soft limits are a little more open to discussion; they are things that you'll approach in certain circumstances, or things that you'd like to work toward over time with trust. You should know your partner's limits and they should know yours. Write them down, if you think that would help. Some people script out a "contract for play" that sets these boundaries. Do whatever makes you feel comfortable so that your boundaries will be respected.

Next up is your safe word. This is an essential part of bondage. A safe word is a word that calls all play to a halt. It signals to participants in a scene that lines have been crossed, and that you are in pain, uncomfortable, unhappy, or distressed. Once the safe word is said, the scene will stop instantly and issues will be addressed. For this reason, your safe word should be quick and easy to remember. I like to use the simple traffic light system: green, yellow, and red, with red being the emergency safe word. It is universal and easy to remember. When one partner is gagged and cannot say his or her safe word, that person should have something small and heavy to drop onto the floor. This action should signal to the top that the submissive wants to stop.

Communication doesn't stop when a scene starts. Good riggers and doms will ensure that communication plays a central role in any bondage scene. You should feel comfortable alerting your top to the fact that the fingers on your left hand have gone tingly. The rigger should deal with the issue before the scene moves on. If at any time you don't feel that you're being properly listened to, bring out your safe word. That's what it's there for, after all. Also it is your responsibility to use that word when you need to. Your partner is not a mind reader. If you need help, say so. You are ultimately responsible for your safety while your partner is there to support you in being safe.

The discussion after a scene is as important as the discussion before it, and it's important to reflect on your experiences honestly. Don't be afraid to say if you didn't particularly enjoy something, or if your needs and desires weren't effectively catered to. Be honest and accepting. This is the key to good communication. It doesn't have to happen right away—enjoy that afterglow! Pick up the conversation when the time is right, but don't wait more than a day. You want the memory to be fresh.

PUSHING BOUNDARIES WITHOUT OVERSTEPPING THEM

We talked about hard and soft limits, and how soft limits can be worked toward or even pushed as part of play. But how do you approach your own limits or someone else's without overstepping boundaries? The truth is that this is difficult, and those who are new to restraint should exercise caution in approaching any limits at all. Play partners should have a history of successful play and should trust each other implicitly before they begin to push the boundaries, and you should never rush into it. Remember: There's always next time.

If you're the dominant in a relationship, start by asking your sub why exactly they want to approach the issues surrounding their soft limits. Some people want to work through self-doubt or trauma while others simply want to experience something they've always been too scared to try. Understanding your bunny's motivation will help you ensure that everyone is satisfied after a scene.

If you're a good top, you'll be constantly on the lookout for any indicators that your sub is uncomfortable or ill at ease, and you will navigate a scene and change tack according to how it's going. When approaching soft limits, it's necessary to be even more attuned to subtle changes in a sub's behavior.

Communicate with your partner during play. It doesn't always have to break a scene; it can be a whisper, a hand signal, or something similar. If you're making a slave beg to be tied and

An experienced partner can take you further than you ever imagined. ▶

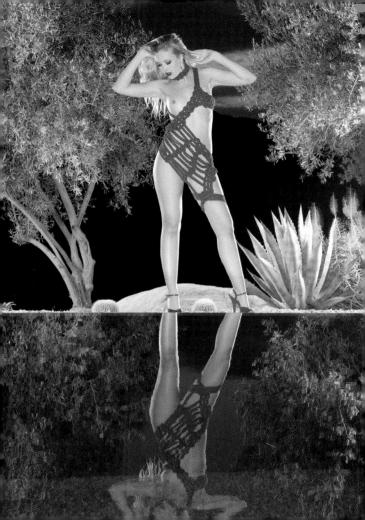

roughed up, you can bring the intensity down for a second to see how calm they become. If he stays agitated, then perhaps you've approached his boundaries enough for one day, and he should be rewarded with something he loves.

THE BASICS OF ROPE SAFETY

All sexual activity has a component of risk, but the physical nature of rope bondage means that you should always keep safety in the back of your mind while you're acting out your devilish fantasies. Ensure that you know whether your partner is prone to panic attacks in certain circumstances. You should also consider getting basic first-aid training.

Of course, the need for information and basic safety care runs through all BDSM—but rope bondage has its own set of safety precautions. The central message of bondage safety is this: You should be able to get your submissive out of any restraint in a matter of seconds.

Rope should never cut into the skin too aggressively, and you should be on the lookout for any indicators of bad circulation or discomfort in your sub. If in doubt about how tight wrist ties are, ask your sub to grab your hand and maintain the grip; if he struggles, the ties need to be loosened. Ties should be snug but loose enough for you to slip one finger in between the skin and the rope. If you're a top, you should always be checking for CSM (circulation, sensation, and movement) in your sub, and if anything seems amiss, undo the ties immediately.

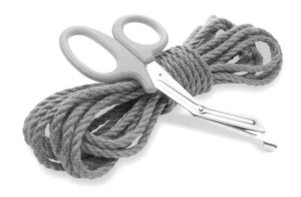

▲ *Safety shears are designed to cut without hurting the skin.*

There is a risk of nerve damage through overextension or compression, where rope presses against a certain area and affects the nerves. This type of damage can take weeks or months to heal, so avoid tying around your submissive's joints or making one area bear too much weight. You should never, ever tie rope around the front of someone's neck.

Good riggers will learn how to tie knots that can be undone quickly, but at some point, it may be necessary to cut your rope, cuffs, duct tape, or other restraint. Keep EMT shears nearby. Bright-color handles make them easier to find. If you prefer metal restraints like chains, locks, and cuffs, invest in a bolt cutter. For handcuffs, keep one key on your regular keychain with your car keys as an extra precaution. Avoid combination locks; it's too easy to forget the code.

No one likes ruining their toys, and if you've just shelled out for a set of gold-plated leg spreaders for your submissive, you aren't exactly going to be thrilled about setting bolt cutters to them. If you expect to think twice about ruining a toy or a rope in an emergency situation, don't buy it. Use more disposable ropes or materials. Nothing is more precious than the health of all those involved, and you'd be surprised what mischief you can get up to with ten dollars' worth of wooden pegs and elastic bands from the convenience store on a Friday night.

You should never, ever leave someone alone when they're restrained. The number one cause of death and serious injury in bondage is someone being alone in restraints. This is nonnegotiable in any circumstance, and if you cannot follow this basic rule of bondage, you should not be playing.

Although a glass of good merlot can loosen you up before a scene and help you let go of your inhibitions, it's never a good idea to be impaired when playing, especially if you're the master or mistress in a session. Impaired thinking is not the friend of safety, so drugs have no place in the bondage dungeon. All partners in all scenes are responsible for the safety of everyone enjoying themselves. Stay sober to avoid threatening the collective safety of the group.

Know the sexual health and history of everyone you play with, and ensure that they know yours. You will get a reputation for bad sexual health in the community if you play fast and loose with this rule. Clean and sterilize all toys, sheets, restraints, surfaces, and floors after a session, and be sure to have a bowl of new condoms, dental dams, and water-based and silicone-based lubes within reach for every scene. Stay safe and sanitary for the sake of all involved.

REMEMBER: CONSENT IS ALWAYS KEY

Consent is affirmative permission given in sound mind.

Read that twice, write it out, and then read it once more. Without consent, there can be no play. Consent is not received by bullying and coercing a partner into letting you do something that you know they don't want to do, whether or not they eventually nod to avoid your constant haranguing or whining. Consent is not given by someone who's drunk or high. Consent is not given if you ignore someone's safe word, or if you simply forgot to bring something up in negotiation and go ahead with it anyway. Without consent, it is abuse.

If you are feeling coerced in the middle of play with things that you previously agreed to, you can simply withdraw your consent by saying "red" and "I don't want to continue, please." It is as simple as that, and your partner will respect it.

Risk-Aware, Consensual Kink (RACK) is the code of conduct in the BDSM world, and for good reason. The most beautiful feeling in bondage is when you can give yourself over to another person, safe in the knowledge that you will be looked after, ravished, and allowed to give in to all your deepest, darkest desires. For us tops, the best thing about kink is to watch a submissive's big eyes look up to you, as the trust shines through even when you're flogging a pair of nice thick buttocks. This cannot be achieved unless consent is soundly obtained.

Don't play with anyone who doesn't value explicit consent, and step in and stop a scene when you believe that one person is abusing another by stepping over set boundaries. Teach by example, and you'll be rewarded with dozens of kinksters lining up to play with you. Who said the good guys never get to have any fun?

Dos and Don'ts

There are a few guidelines to follow when exploring rope bondage.

DON'T:

- *Leave someone in bondage alone.*
- *Let rope cut into the body.*
- *Make ties too tight.*
- *Tie anything around the throat.*
- *Buy anything that you won't be comfortable cutting off someone in an emergency.*
- *Approach hard limits.*
- *Drink or take drugs before playtime.*
- *Play with a partner who you don't trust 100 percent.*
- *Ignore someone's discomfort.*
- *Coerce partners into doing something outside of their comfort zone.*

DO:

- *Obtain consent.*
- *Know the health history, sexual and otherwise, of any play partners.*
- *Warm up before a scene.*
- *Always have EMT shears, bolt cutters, and first-aid equipment nearby.*
- *Check for CSM throughout a bondage scene.*
- *Engage in good negotiation and communication throughout a session.*
- *Approach soft limits with caution.*
- *Be clean and sanitary.*
- *Practice safe sex.*
- *Set a safe word.*
- *Have fun playing, but take safety seriously.*

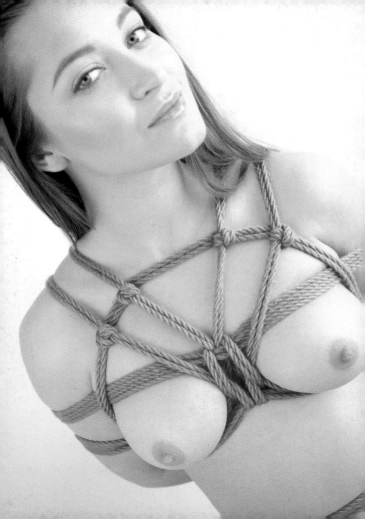

Chapter 3

THE EQUIPMENT— KNOW YOUR ROPE

Bondage equipment doesn't have to strain your wallet. If your bondage budget only gets you an old rope and two rolls of duct tape, don't worry: You're going to have just as much fun with those two materials as you could with 100 meters of neon rope. Bondage is all about your perverted mind. Toys and materials are just the different tools you use to make those kinky dreams into reality.

In this chapter, we'll discuss all kinds of rope and other materials that you can use for bondage, but don't be put off by the seemingly endless arsenal of equipment listed; you don't need it all. You may be surprised at what you can get for cheap at the convenience store.

Although many materials can be used to restrict or tie someone, rope is the preferred material of many, thanks to its resilience, ease of use, and versatility. It's a sex toy that doesn't require batteries, doesn't involve a lot of preparation time, doesn't get your fingers all covered in lube, and doesn't shock your family if someone finds it in a drawer.

DIFFERENT TYPES OF ROPE

There are many types of rope, but not all are suitable for rope bondage. Though it might seem tempting to just grab that dusty pile of rope that's been sitting in the garage for almost twenty years and start tying your husband up with it, let's first look at the different ropes available and why we use them.

Bondage ropes can be lumped into two basic categories: natural and synthetic. Natural fiber ropes are made of materials such as jute, hemp, and linen. These materials are very hardy and are twisted rather than braided. They also tend to be rough against the skin, especially hemp, so rope makers treat the fibers by boiling and then oiling them to make them smooth. Jute is naturally more supple and smooth than hemp, and linen, though gorgeous to touch, is the least often used. The biggest benefit of using any of these types of natural-fiber ropes is that their knot-holding ability exceeds that of synthetic-fiber ropes, with jute in particular being up to just about any task you could think of. For this reason, jute has been traditionally used for *shibari*.

The most popular natural fiber for ropes is cotton. Unlike other types of natural-fiber rope, cotton rope can be braided as well as twisted, which makes it a lot easier on the skin. However, cotton rope isn't as strong as other natural-fiber ropes, and the lack of friction from the material can mean that knots are more likely to slip out. Still, the wide availability and affordability of cotton, as well as its softness against skin and general ease of use, make it a great choice for many nonsuspension ties and binds. Almost all the colored rope in this book is cotton with some bamboo thrown in. You should be able to find cotton rope at home improvement and craft stores, and it won't break the bank.

Synthetic fibers are also popular, and nylon is the number one material for bondage rope. Nylon is relatively cheap, widely available, smooth, and will keep its shape when knotted into beautiful ties, unlike other materials. It's also easily wiped clean. More important, it's always easy to untie and won't terrify new bondage partners like untreated hemp will. The only catch is you have to pick it up before you buy it. The softer it feels, the better it will be against your rope bunny's skin.

Parachute cord and thick yarn are synthetics that can be used for bondage, but both are thin and relatively weak. They are suitable for decorative knots or for use on smaller body parts. You can use parachute cord to tie fingers together or to bind genitals. Because cord and yarn are cheap, you can cut them off and throw them away when you are done.

Dedicated riggers and rope bunnies will often have a collection of ropes made from different materials. My personal favorites are cotton, jute, hemp, and then nylon. Nylon is a great go-to, all-purpose rope when you are just getting started because it is strong and cheap compared with others. You can dye it with fabric dye, and the gorgeous shades that you can get mean that your playtime will always be beautiful. You can hit up local artists that hand-make rope like I do, or others that process and soften the rope so it is ready for use with people.

As well as in material, ropes also differ in length and diameter, and unless you want to find yourself halfway through a harness tie with no rope left to finish it, it's important to make note of which lengths are used for which types of ties. In terms of length, anything from 5 feet (1.5 m) to 60 feet (18 m) can be used in rope bondage. At the shorter end, you can find length perfect for limb bondage, while the longer ropes will allow you to tie beautiful harness ties and suspension rigs. If you're into shibari, you'll want to get some lengths cut to about 25 feet (7.6 m) or 30 feet (9 m) each, but once you've found your way through the basic bondage ties, there's really no wrong length of rope. In terms of diameter of rope to use, I prefer between ¼ and ⅜ of an inch (6 mm and 1 cm) and about 30 feet (9 m) long. Rope that's thicker than ½ inch (1.3 cm) can be difficult to use and won't allow you to make the beautiful ties that you crave to see on your supple sub.

Throughout this book you will see the natural-fiber rope doubled over and used as one line. This is so the rope can go on twice as fast, and if you need to split directions, you can. There are certain conventions we use for rope bondage, with the 30 foot (9 m)-length being one of the most consistent. But remember: Rope is just a tool. It is the mind that makes it art.

TOOLS FOR YOUR BEDSIDE DRAWER

Whether you're into rope bondage for sex, the bedroom is a comfortable and private place for rigging your partner. Make sure that your toy drawer is always stocked with the correct equipment to keep your bondage time safe and sexy.

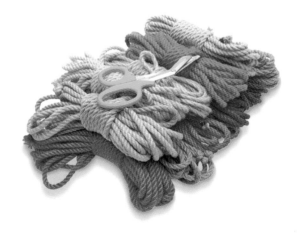

▲ *Rope comes in many types and colors—as do these essential safety shears.*

As previously mentioned, whenever you engage in even light bondage, you should have EMT shears within reach at all times, as well as a first aid kit, blankets, and all the other safety equipment we've discussed. Rescue hooks can also be a great investment, as they are easier to use than safety shears and will always get your sub out of a tie immediately. Never play alone.

Arnica cream, body cream, condoms, dental dams, and different types of lube should always be nearby during playtime, as well as any sex toys that you might want to experiment with. Remember: Safety is always key!

NONROPE TOYS AND MATERIALS

You can use almost anything to tie a person up—wool to tie his fingers, a beach towel to mummify him, or a necktie to bind her hands to the bedframe. I have some favorite nonrope materials for any scene or playtime.

The least intimidating materials are things that you might usually find in the bedroom, such as neckties, scarves, belts, and pairs of tights or stockings. One of my favorite moves involves a pillowcase: turn your submissive over, pull the sub's arms together behind his or her back, make your sub grab his or her elbows, and simply pull the pillowcase up over his or her arms. It's simple, but effective!

Duct tape is a great material for bondage as you always have some in the house, but if you love the idea of restriction without tearing your arm hair out, try bondage tape. It is especially made for our purposes and isn't coated with any adhesive; it only sticks to itself. The useful thing about bondage tape is that, as well as coming in an array of beautiful colors, it's reusable and can be wiped clean. For a budget-friendly option with a similar effect, use plastic wrap, but be careful not to wrap anyone's rib cage too tightly. My favorite way to use plastic wrap is to bind legs so that they're bent back under themselves; this way, your submissive is immobilized but you can still move them around to put them in different positions. Cutting them out when you're finished is also fun.

There are a lot of different premade bondage toys available. In fact, there are probably more than you could ever use in a whole lifetime (although I've given it a damn good go, believe me). Collars and cuffs are favorites among the bondage crowd, as these tend to be beautifully made, comfortable, great-looking, and easy to use. For instance, you can buy a silk-lined black leather collar for your submissive as a gift for good behavior, and the small clasp on the front will allow you to attach a rope or chain to it and walk her around the house like a housebroken puppy. The same goes for wrist and ankle cuffs. These toys are made by perverts, for perverts, so they know exactly what you want to use them for and manufacture them accordingly.

What NOT to Use

Although it's important to know which type of rope to use in what situation, it's absolutely imperative to understand when you simply cannot use a rope or other material. This is an issue of safety, and therefore should be at the forefront of your mind in any scene. Using the wrong material in the wrong situation can be incredibly dangerous, so ensure that you understand these restrictions.

Polypropylene ropes are used for outdoor activities such as water-skiing. It is a rough rope to the touch. No one wants that sort of chafing when they're trying to get into the zone. Polypropylene ropes are also hard to work with and don't tend to hold knots very well, making them unsafe for any sort of suspension ties. Having your submissive wriggle free because the rope is no good can also kill a scene, so avoid this type of rope entirely.

Climbing rope is about as expensive as it is gorgeous. Climbers, like kinksters, aren't afraid to drop some serious money to get high-quality, attractive equipment. Climbing rope is strong and durable, but it's too thick and makes knots that are far too big and bulky.

Natural fibers such as coir, sisal, and manila are rough on the skin and difficult to work with. If you enjoy the feeling of a rougher rope against your flesh, I recommend using hemp rope over any of these three.

You might think an authentic pair of handcuffs would be fun to restrain your submissive with. The truth is that they are not. Handcuffs are designed specifically to be harsh, uncomfortable, and difficult to get out of, meaning that if your poor partner struggles even a little bit, the metal will cut into the sensitive parts of his wrists and even get caught around his wristbones in odd ways. The worst thing about handcuffs is losing the keys. They're too small, especially when you're both wriggling around, and you'll end up searching under the bed for an hour while your partner sits there bored and desperately needing to pee. There are many other ways to tie your partner's wrists to your bedframe, so leave the handcuffs for the cops.

We discussed duct tape earlier, and this can be one of the easiest and most fun ways to restrain someone on the fly. However, you should never wrap tape around someone's neck or nostrils, and if you bind them too tightly in a nonbreathable material around their torso, they won't have space to breathe properly. Never let yourself get too carried away with duct tape, electrical tape, gaffer tape, or whatever other tape you have laying around the house. Safety always comes first.

BASIC ROPE BONDAGE KIT

If you're just starting out in bondage and don't want to invest too much time or money searching for the right types of rope only to realize that you've got nowhere to hide your purchases, then your basic bondage equipment might just be a scarf and an old tie. There's no reason that you can't play around with the concept of restraint using simple items. However, if this type of play turns you on in a way that makes you want to go further, now's the time to invest in some rope and a few leg spreaders—but remember not to buy anything that you won't feel comfortable cutting through or breaking to release a panicking sub!

Here are a few things that I would consider necessary for any self-respecting rope bondage lover.

Beginner Rope Bondage Bag:

- *EMT shears*
- *2 pieces of 30-foot (9 m) rope, ¼ inch (6 mm) diameter*
- *1 silk scarf*

Intermediate Rope Bondage Bag:

- *EMT shears*
- *6 pieces of 30-foot (9 m) rope, ¼ inch (6 mm) diameter*
- *2 carabineers*
- *1 men's necktie*

Serious Rope Bondage Bag:

- *EMT shears*
- *12 pieces of 30-foot (9 m) rope, ¼ inch (6 mm) diameter*
- *4 pieces of 15-foot (4.6 m) rope, ¼ inch (6 mm) diameter*
- *2 pieces of 15-foot (4.6 m), $^5/_{32}$ inch (4 mm) diameter*
- *2 carabineers*
- *1 suspension ring*
- *Scarves and men's ties*
- *Bondage tape*
- *3 leather belts*

Put your rope away nice and neat for next time. ▶

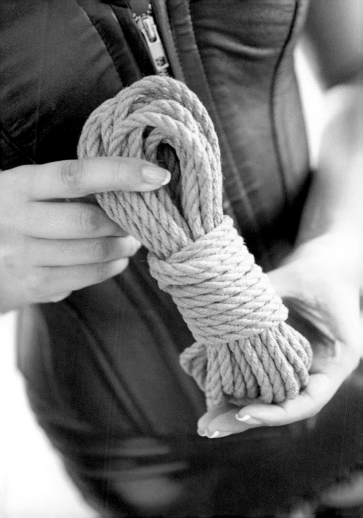

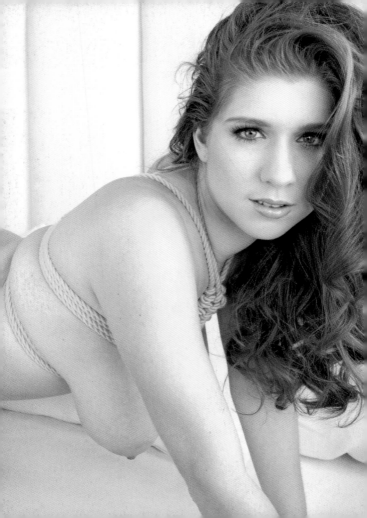

Chapter 4

CHOOSING YOUR BONDAGE PARTNER

Remember in high school when your teacher would announce that it was time for group work and everyone would let out a collective groan? Thankfully, we're all grown adults now, and most of the time, we get to pick who we play with. However, with all the joy of this decision comes responsibility too. No one's going to drop the perfect play partner into your lap, all trussed up and ready to go with a brand-new rope thrown in for good measure. It's up to you to find a kinky person who loves to be tied up in rope and has all the physical and mental strength that you seek in a rope bunny.

EMOTIONAL STABILITY

What do you look for in a play partner? Bondage can bring up a lot of intense feelings and emotions—for the rigger as well as the person who's bound—and you want to be able to process these feelings with a partner.

If you're an experienced and well-respected rigger, you'll have rope bunnies lining up at your door, in which case it's up to them to prove to you that they'll be fantastic play partners. However, if you're just getting into bondage, it can be a little more difficult to find someone suitable, especially if you don't know what you should be looking for.

First think of all the things that you look for in a friend. You'll want someone you like to spend time with. Do you like your friends to have a sense of humor, and do you like to feel comfortable and at ease in their presence? Most likely it follows that these are the traits you should look for in a play partner. Look for someone trustworthy, fun, and willing to talk about his or her bondage history, sexual and mental health, and what he or she really wants out of your playtime. Look for someone who's open and engaging and without drama.

You should also look for a partner who's emotionally stable and lucid. This isn't to say that you can't play with others who have experienced trauma or difficulty in their lives or those who have emotional sore spots. If your potential rope bunny has obvious issues that he or she is hiding or refuses to address, politely say no. Rope bondage is often an intense experience, and you should be sure that any potential partner will be able to experience it in a safe and respectful way.

If you're a rope bunny looking for a top, the same goes. Be thorough when meeting with a potential dominant, and don't go a step further than talking until you're sure that you can trust that person. Outline your hard boundaries, desires, experience, and health, and ask about your partner's. Try to ascertain what type of person he or she is, and if, even for a second, that person makes you feel uncomfortable, politely say no and end the meeting. Ensure that you meet any potential top in a public place the first time and that a friend knows where you are. Remember that this person will be in total control of your health and well-being, and don't be afraid to be picky. The right top is always worth the wait!

NEWBIES VS. EXPERIENCED PARTNERS

You may be relatively new to the world of rope bondage. You might be exploring with someone who is just as inexperienced as you, or you might meet someone who has been in the scene for a long time. This makes a huge impact on how your first steps into bondage will go—and, of course, how quickly you can get to the really kinky stuff! If your partner is also new to bondage, then you'll want to take things slowly. The world of bondage is expansive and there's no need to rush to the finish line. If you've never tied anyone, start with something light—duct tape around the wrists, maybe. Try ravishing, caressing, and teasing, before turning your partner over and taking him or her like you've paid for it. Try different positions and roles to see which fits you. Build up slowly, being sure not to push your partner too far. When you finally play with rope, try the simplest ties first. After your first rope session, allow for an extended aftercare period, as rope can bring out some severe reactions at first, and don't dive right back into it if your partner needs a little recovery time. Don't forget that there's no shame in saying you don't like something.

If you're lucky enough to have an experienced bondage friend, partner, teacher, or top, then your road into bondage will be a little smoother, although not altogether dissimilar. When I play with a bondage virgin, we first sit down and talk in a public place. We'll chat about our histories, experiences, and what we both wish to get from the encounter. Once we're both comfortable and excited to play with each other, we'll plan a date for our first play session. I'll make sure that my new bunny is relaxed and sober, and that my toys don't look too scary or intimidating. I'll use a soft rope, such as cotton or hemp, that is less challenging than scratchy jute, and we'll play around a little beforehand. Only when the bunny is mentally and physically ready will we start with some easy, comfy ties. If you're introducing a beginner bunny to bondage, start with the ties in chapter 6. From the first conversation to the final rigging session, we will only ever go as quickly as the bunny wants to.

HEALTH

Whether you're getting started in rope bondage with a new partner, or starting to tie up the man you've been married to for thirty years, going over the health history of all interested parties is a necessity before rope is even uncoiled. Sit down together and list every health issue you have or have ever had, and ensure that your partner has a copy of this list. This is especially important for those who are playing with new partners. Include any emotional issues in this list as well. And don't worry—if you have joint problems or heart trouble, it doesn't mean that you can't have a fulfilling exploration into bondage. Even the terminally inflexible with rope allergies can have a tantalizing bondage life.

Though you might know your partner inside out (quite literally) once you've tied each other up a few times, remember that it's always important to check how your partner is feeling before a session. Your bunny might have pulled a muscle in the gym or might have not slept very well, meaning that she isn't as strong as usual. Take it easy during this session.

It's never easy to ask, "When was your last HIV test?" during a warm, intimate encounter with a potential bondage partner, but it's one of the questions you need to ask before you begin playing. Only you can be responsible for your sexual health; don't let others do it for you. You should be upfront about it, and so should your partner. Don't trust a person who brushes off a question. If someone isn't transparent about their sexual past, don't play with them. You should also consider that the nature of sexually transmitted infections is that a person (including you) may not even know that he or she has one, so regular checks are essential if you're planning to have a diverse and exciting sexual life. And always remember: Play safe!

THE POWER PLAY

The exchange of power is at the crux of all BDSM. For a top, the feeling of having a person give their liberty over to you entirely is heavenly; for a bottom, giving their power over to another for a short session allows them to experience great pleasure. For a rope bunny, being bound brings feelings of freedom, euphoria, sexual fulfillment, and joy. For a rigger, being in total control of another brings the same feelings.

All this exciting sexiness can occur because of a thick layer of trust padding any hypothetical sharp edges. Without trust, bondage can be difficult and painful. But how do you know that you're going to be totally comfortable exchanging power with a potential partner?

No matter how hot and heavy the action gets, safety should be at the forefront of your mind. ▶

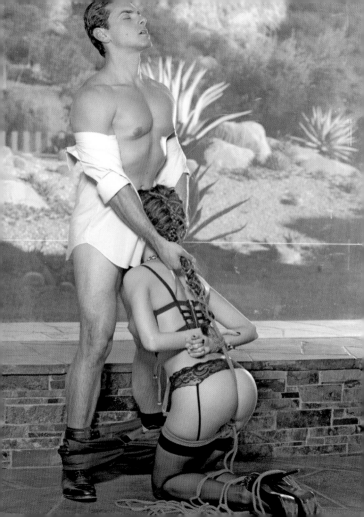

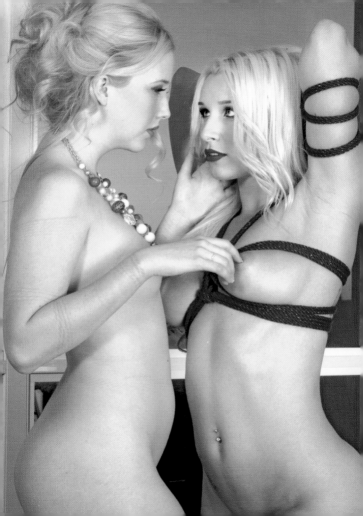

One great way to figure out how you're going to feel in a power play with someone is to let that person blindfold you and guide you around a public or private place. Go to a fetish- or BDSM-themed event with your potential top, who will have control over you for a little while. Your top should help you ease into the situation, then slip the blindfold over your eyes and tie a piece of string (gently) to your wrist. Let him or her guide you around, while taking the utmost care to describe what's around you and make sure you don't bump into anything. If it's working, you'll feel a little embarrassed but a little turned on; if it's not, you'll feel awkward and kind of anxious. Try switching roles and see if that's better. If not, maybe that partner just isn't for you. Don't worry—there are plenty more kinky fish in the bondage sea!

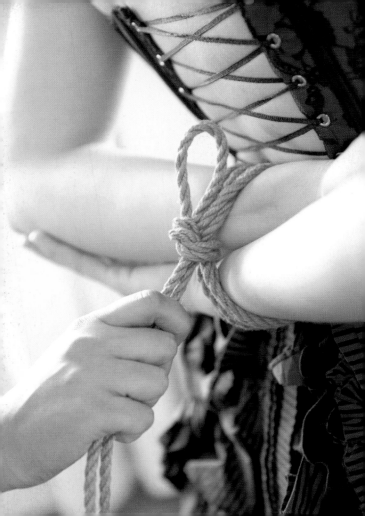

Chapter 5

BASIC KNOTS

By now, you should be ready to properly begin your journey into bondage. First riggers need to learn basic knots before creating full-body bondage ties. Not only will tying an exquisite body harness make you look like a bit of a newbie if you don't have the basics down, but it can also be dangerous. If you place supporting knots in places they shouldn't go, you can injure your sub. Pushing yourself to become better is encouraged—but it's important to appreciate your own limitations when someone's safety is literally in your hands.

Learn and practice these basic knots: They are your bondage alphabet. Some of you have been lucky enough to be Boy Scouts, sailors, or climbers. For the sake of the total newbies, I'm assuming a prior knowledge of zero—and even if you think you know these knots by heart, it won't hurt to refresh your memory.

BULA BULA

This is a classic knot that is the most basic one for starting your ties. It is easy and quick to learn and apply.

1. Begin by folding your rope in half. Next, take the middle part of your rope and wrap it around the wrist or ankle three times.

2. After completing the wraps, cross both ends perpendicularly.

3. The wraps should be loose enough that you can tuck the short end under the wraps and hook it with your thumb and pull through.

4. Make a loop on the other end in the direction you see here.

5. Pull the short (bight) end through.

6. Tighten the whole knot. This knot has the advantage of being tied quickly and efficiently but is not recommended for rope bondage suspension.

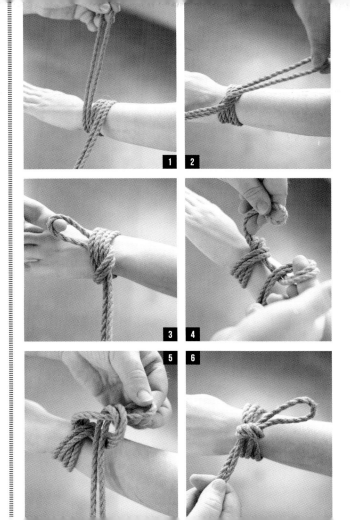

LARK'S HEAD KNOT

This is a kind of constriction knot because the harder you pull it, the tighter it gets. It is one of the most basic knots and will help you get into artistic rope bondage easily.

1. Take the middle of the rope in a loop. We call this loop the bight end.

2. Wrap it around your thumb and pull the long end through.

3. Just like this! This knot can then be slipped over the ends of the rope (coming up in a moment) or be tied in the middle of a rope when you need a tight knot that won't slide around.

4. Here's what the other side of the knot looks like.

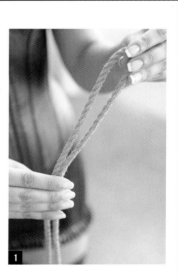

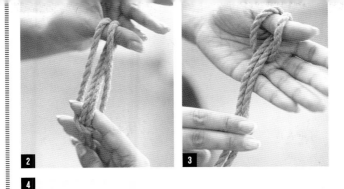

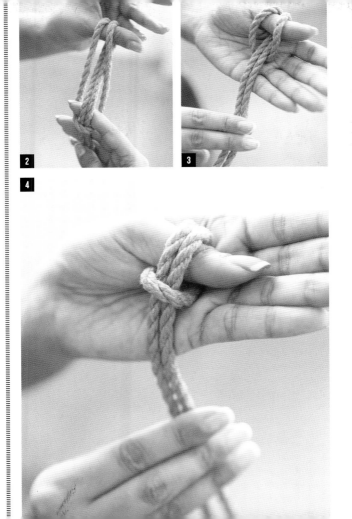

THE MUNTER HITCH

This knot is used mostly for decorative crossovers and changes of direction. You have to keep steady pressure on the knot while tying it or else it falls apart. It makes your ties look more polished when crossing rope than if you just loop around.

1. Start with the bight end and another piece of rope you want to cross over. Here, our model has a chest harness already tied, and we want to add another piece of rope to carry on a more decorative element. Cross the bight end perpendicularly over the other rope.

2. Bring the loop (bight) end under the rope you are crossing.

3. Now bring it across and over the end of the same piece of rope you are using.

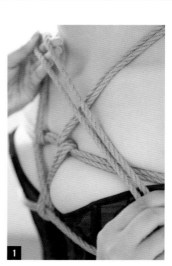

4. Cross back under the rope you just tied around and carry on with the rest of your rope bondage.

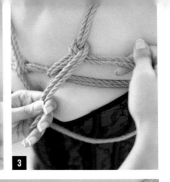

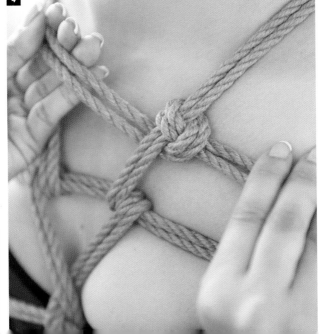

SOMMERVILLE BOWLINE

This knot is a unidirectional knot that is great for starting intermediate ties.

1. Start by grasping your length of rope in the middle and then wrap it around your partner's wrist three times. It doesn't have to be tight—in fact, a little slack is best.

2. Once you have the wraps completed, take the ends and cross them perpendicularly.

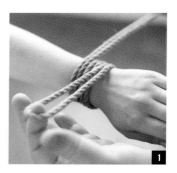

3. Holding the short (bight) end, wrap the long end around it in the direction you see here. It is important that the wrap is in the correct direction.

4. Here is the tricky part—push two fingers through the large loop you just made and under all the wraps around the wrist.

5. Bend the short end backward and grasp it with the fingers

that you just pushed through the loop. Now pull that end back through the loop.

6. Now start to tighten the whole knot evenly.

7. Once it is all snug, you should have a rope "cuff" that won't constrict on the wrist. The bonus of this knot is that it holds in all directions and is easy to untie.

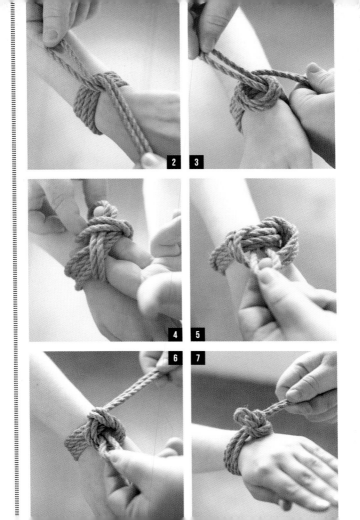

WRISTS BEHIND

This is the only time we tie wrists without any rope in between the wrists. It is because this tie doesn't have to be so tight it cuts off any circulation.

1. Start by having your partner fold their arms behind their back. Wrap the bight end around both wrists, as shown.

2. Cross the bight end perpendicularly so that the rope has changed direction and is in line with the way the arms are laying.

3. Take the loop end and tuck it through the natural opening created by the arms folded together and gently but firmly snug the tie down.

4. Make an overhand knot against this whole bundle.

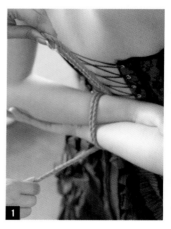

5. The knot should look exactly like this. When your partner's arms are like this, take care to make sure your partner can maintain their balance.

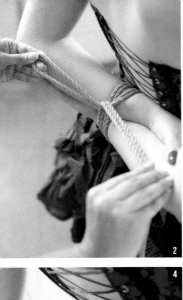

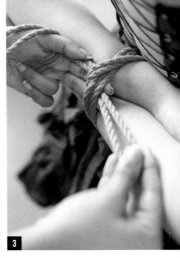

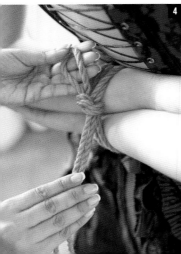

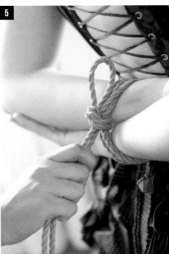

TWO-COLUMN TIE

This can be used for any "two columns" you encounter, such as your partner's wrists.

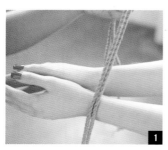
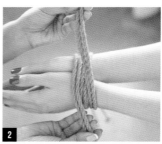

1. Start with the bight end (the loop) and have your lover bring his or her arms together. They don't have to be tight, because there will be rope in between them when you are done.

2. Wrap the rope around the wrists a few times.

3. Now, cross the rope and change direction.

4. Drop the loop end down between the wrists and wrap it under and back up so you come up in the center of the arms.

5. Tie an overhand knot.

6. Tie one more knot on top of that.

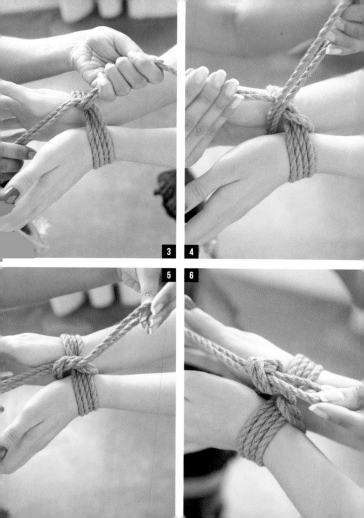

TIE

Use this comfortable and easy tie when you want to cross the wrists.

1. Start by making a few wraps around the wrists, keeping the wraps flat with no twists.

2. Cross the rope at the base of the thumb.

3. Wrap between the wrists.

4. Come all the way back down and get ready to cross the free end of the rope.

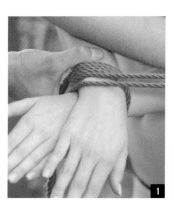

5. Make a nice, easy knot right here. Tip: Keep the knot in an easy-to-get-at place like the underside of the arms, not in between the wrists.

6. This finished tie can also be used to bind the ankles.

7. The simplicity of this tie means you can get creative with positions! Try throwing your partner over your shoulders for a little reward.

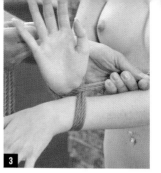

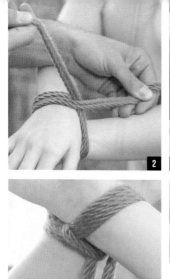

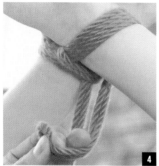

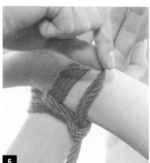

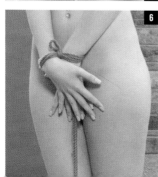

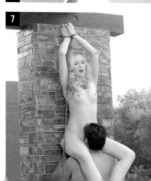

NECKTIE SEX HARNESS

Instead of rope, this hip harness uses neckties to bind your partner, with handles for you to grab on to. You can even use long scarves—the knots and pattern are the same.

1. Capture your beauty around the waist, right in the middle of the tie.

2. Make a simple knot over one hip.

3. Wrap the back end of the tie up between the legs and the front end down between the legs to the back. Make sure the tie lies flat, not twisted.

4. Come back up and retie a new knot over top of the original one.

5. Repeat with another tie on the other side, making the knots comfortable but not loose.

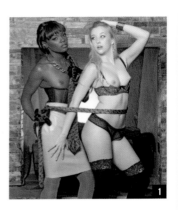

6. It should look the same on both sides. Don't forget to tuck in your ends.

7. You can complete almost any tie in this book with enough neckties!

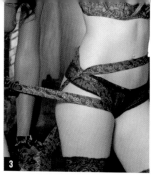

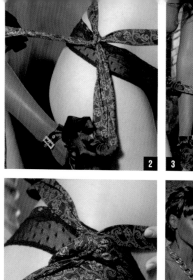

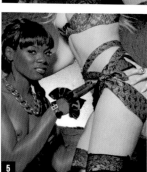

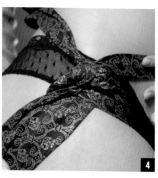

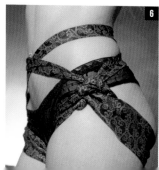

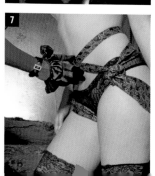

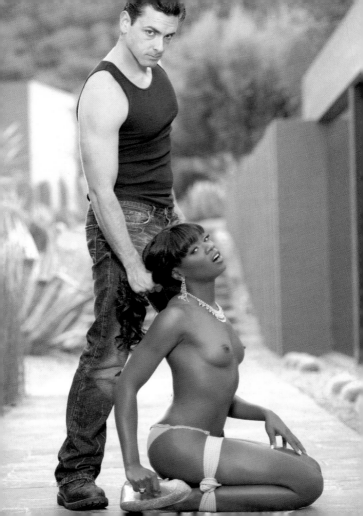

Chapter 6

THE TIES

You should be itching to move on to the next level of your rope bondage adventure. We'll start off with some basic ties to use on one body part; this way, you can progress to tying your partner's wrists to your metal bedframe. You'll see that there are variations of many of the ties—a way to go a little further, or to turn that upper-body tie into a full-body tie. You should practice these separately and together. Of course, the poses suggested here are just the tip of the iceberg; I'll let your filthy mind do the rest of the work.

NOVICE HAIR TIE

This tie is more secure and works well with longer hair, as you will braid the rope all the way through it.

1. Start by taking the middle of the rope and make an overhand knot around the base of the ponytail.

2. Take the loop and start to tuck it down through the hair above the base of the ponytail, against the head.

3. Lift up the ponytail and pull it all the way through, leaving about 1½ inches (4 cm) below.

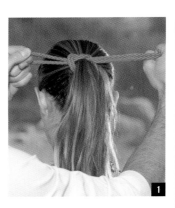

4. Now feed the free end of the rope through the loop and snug it up.

5. Gather the hair into three sections, put the two pieces of rope into two sections, and start braiding.

6. Braid all the way to the end, then form a large loop and pull it through.

7. Tighten it at the bottom and enjoy.

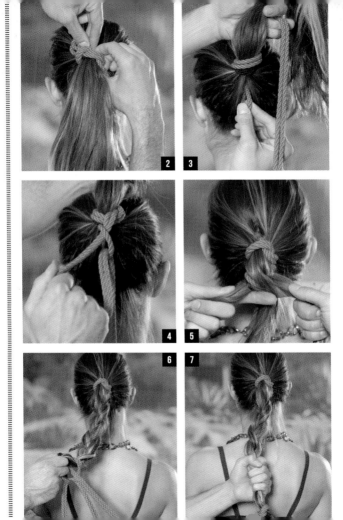

ADVANCED HAIR TIE

This hair tie looks prettier and will hold about as well as the Novice Hair Tie.

1. Start by pushing the loop up from the bottom, behind the hair elastic.

2. Bring the long end of the rope up over the hair and feed it through loop. This will form a secure base.

3. Now make a loop with the free end on the inside of the loop.

4. Pull it tight. The form of this turn in the rope will hold it in place.

5. Repeat all the way down.

6. When you get to the end, finish it off with an overhand knot up against the last turn in the rope.

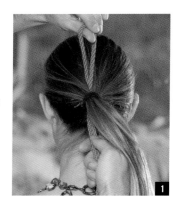

7. It looks long and neat, ready for a night out.

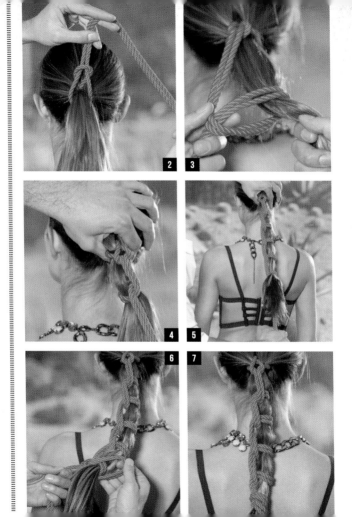

KNEELING TWO-COLUMN LEG TIE

This is an easy tie for getting your partner into a comfortable and proper kneeling position and keeping them there. It has a nice wide band across the leg, which makes it more comfortable.

1. Have your partner kneel and make three wraps around his or her leg. Keep the wraps up near the thigh, allowing space between the foot and leg.

2. Finish the wrapping so you have about 14 inches (35.5 cm) left of the loop end. Cross it with the free end.

3. Now take the free end, tuck it down, and wrap it around the other wraps on the other side.

4. Pull it up again and cinch it tight. Finish this as a Bula Bula (page 54).

5. Push the loop over the final free end and cinch it down a second time.

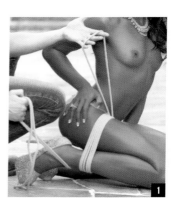

6. Tuck all your ends in.

7. Finish with your partner kneeling at your feet.

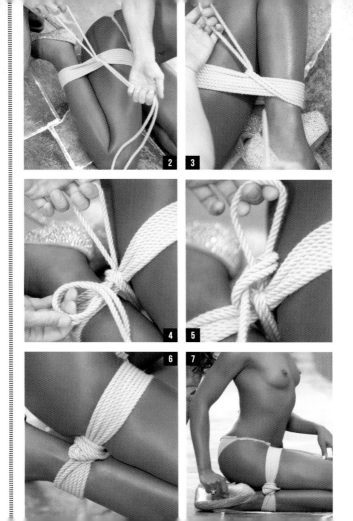

SIMPLE STRAPPADO

To add a more forceful element, a simple arm binder is effective at keeping your partner in place.

1. Begin with a Two-Column Tie (page 64) around the wrists.

2. Bring the rope up vertically and wrap it around her upper arms above the elbows. Keep tension on the rope.

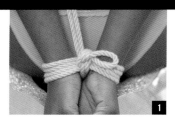

3. When the wraps are on, pass the rope around the middle, like you did with the kneeling tie. Pick up the wraps on the other side and gently pull the arms together at the elbow and cinch it down. Tip: Not everyone's body can do this. Your partner can raise her elbows upward for more room and flexibility.

4. Take the rope and come over the left shoulder. Drop the rope down and through the left armpit and bring it across the back.

5. Come up through the right armpit, over the right shoulder, and back to the cinch where the elbows are trapped.

6. Finish the tie neatly.

7. Now your partner is completely under your control. You can lift the arms gently Tip: Having your partner bend forward will lift her arms and make the position feel more submissive. Go slowly and gently. You want a sexy stretch, not a painful one.

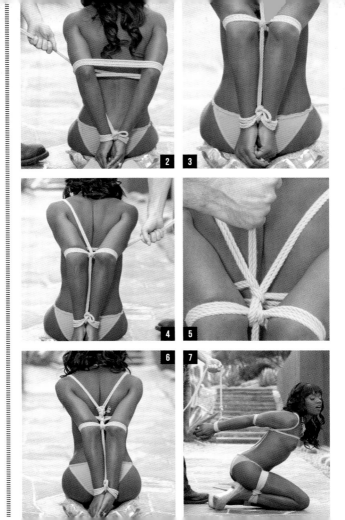

MEN'S CHEST HARNESS

This is an intermediate chest tie that takes only one length of rope and a followed pattern to pull it together. This chest harness is designed to accentuate a masculine chest and keep your man's arms firmly behind his back.

1. Capture the wrists using the Wrists Behind tie (page 62) and come up over the right shoulder and then down through the armpit to the back.

2. Come across the back, up through the left armpit and over the left shoulder, and then back to the center.

3. Make just a few wraps to keep it all in place.

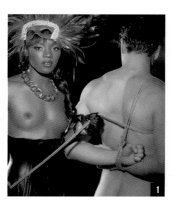

4. Come up through the right armpit again, across the chest, and pull it through the left shoulder rope.

5. Come back and under the right shoulder rope.

6. Form a quick Munter Hitch

(page 58) and go across the chest and through the left armpit to the back and tie it off.

7. Now that he's restrained, it's time to take control. It takes a strong man to be in this kind of rope!

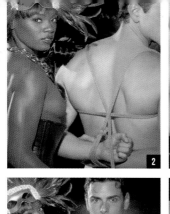

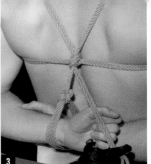

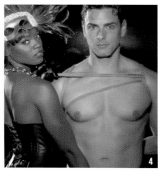

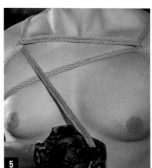

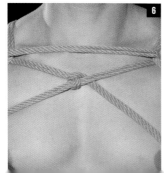

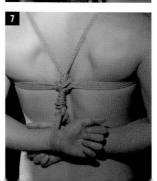

BASIC FUTO

This is a basic beginning to a great Futo tie (a Western name for a Japanese bondage standard). It is more complicated than the simple Two-Column Tie (page 64) but it looks very pretty and is more comfortable.

1. Start with a simple Bula Bula (page 54) or Sommerville Bowline (page 60) around the ankle.

2. Wrap from the bottom upward, keeping the lower leg pushed against the thigh.

3. Make four wraps and then bring a final half wrap around to catch the top horizontal wrap.

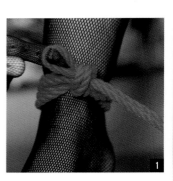

4. Make a simple overhand wrap around each horizontal and work your way downward.

5. Once you reach the bottom, tuck it under the last wrap and through. Bend her leg forward so you can work your way upward on the outside.

6. If you have a lot of rope left, retrace your steps, building a new layer, coming back through and up the inside, wrapping in a twisting motion around all the verticals.

7. Enjoy your partner all tied up with legs spread.

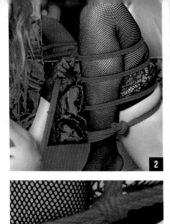

2

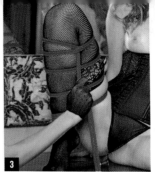

3

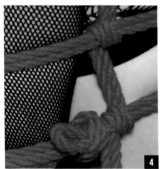

4

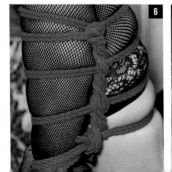

5

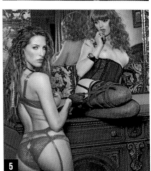

6

7

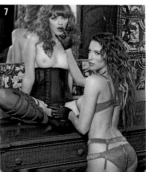

LADDER TIE

Now that we've mastered the arm binder, let's move on to binding the legs! This is a great tie for a rope bunny who likes to feel helpless and completely bound.

1. First, tie the ankles with a simple Two-Column Tie (page 64).

2. Come around the back with the rope and make two wraps around the shins.

3. Tuck the rope up and over the wraps on the other side of the vertical rope.

4. You don't have to tie a knot in the back if you can keep the tension on the rope. Come between the legs and up over the shin wraps.

5. Come back through and make a wrap around the vertical rope again.

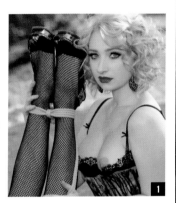

6. Repeat all the way up the body, making wraps every 10 inches (25 cm). Tie just below and above the knees—not right on the joint.

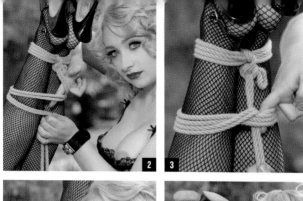

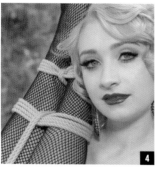

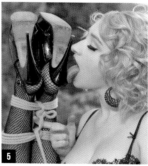

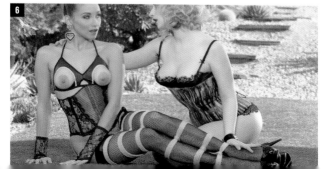

ASYMMETRIC CHEST TIE FOR MEN

This tie is fun, strong, and when tied over clothes that are later pulled open, looks super sexy. All the main knots are in the back.

1. Start with his hands tied behind his back in a Two-Column Tie (page 64) and then wrap his chest and shoulder above his nipples.

2. Wrap twice around the chest and shoulders and then, on the right side, come up between his arm and chest and over the shoulder. Then pull the rope down under his left armpit and across the front.

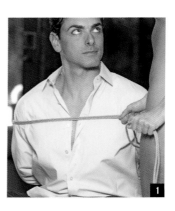

3. Go back the way you came. Your neat set of wraps should pull on the vertical rope over his right shoulder.

4. You're in charge! Bend him over and hold him in place as you finish the ties in the back.

5. Carry the free end of the rope and pull up the lower wrap.

6. Tuck it under, cinch it tight, and then finish with a knot in the back.

7. Be a good boy and do everything that the wicked lady tells you to!

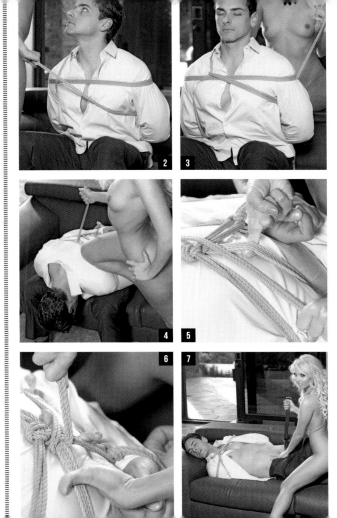

SEXY SELF-TIED CHEST HARNESS

No one says you have to have your partner tie you up! You can do it by yourself. However, it's good practice to have a partner and safety scissors nearby.

1. Start with a simple loop around the chest, under the breasts.

2. Come through the loop and reverse around the way you just came, back around the chest.

3. Pull the rope through your original loop.

4. Take the rope up between the breasts, hold it in place while you change direction, and make a wrap around the chest above the breasts. Tip: Keep tension on the rope as you do this.

5. Make another double pass around the chest, above the breasts. Come back through the loop you just created.

6. You can get creative with tying it off. Make a pair of

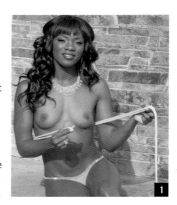

diagonal passes with the rope. Then pass the rope around to the back of the body.

7. To finish, you can loop the rope around your shoulders, pass it down to the vertical rope at your chest, and use a simple weaving back and forth to finish the ends.

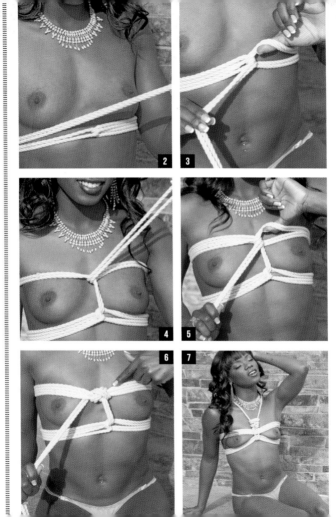

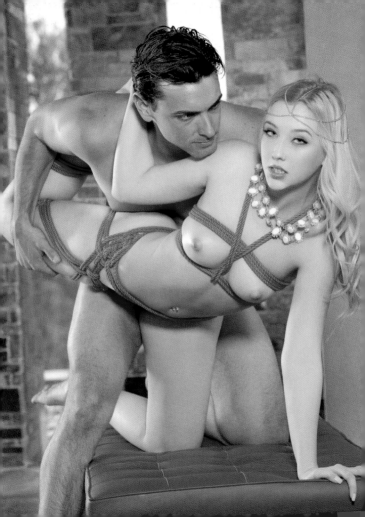

Chapter 7

TAKING IT FURTHER

By now, you should be feeling a lot more confident wielding a nice bit of rope. Now you can piece together your knowledge of the basics to form intermediate ties and create new works of art. In this chapter, you'll see how some binds can be extended to form full-torso harnesses or to allow you to tie arms and legs together at the same time. You'll see that basically all the more intermediate ties are built upon the same foundations that we practiced in chapter 5.

There's nothing more scintillating than binding your sub in intricate arrangements and seeing her eyes silently beg you for more. These harnesses are perfect for having your filthy way with someone.

SIMPLE CHEST HARNESS FOR WOMEN

This is a great, simple chest harness to start because it will act as a foundation for adding onto later.

1. Begin by pulling the rope around the body and back through the loop (or bight, the middle of the rope).

2. Come over the shoulder and down the middle, crossing over and under, then back up again over the opposite shoulder.

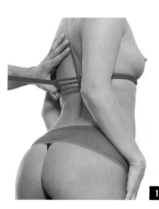

3. Pull the rope over the right shoulder and bring it under the horizontal wrap. Pull it up between the wrap and the base of the left shoulder rope and make a simple knot to hold it secure.

4. Come around the front, under the arm, and pull the rope from under and then inside to out. Form a Munter Hitch knot (page 58) here.

5. Complete a hitch on the opposite side.

6. Tie it off in back.

7. If you have any rope left over, drop a length down and bundle up your partner's wrists.

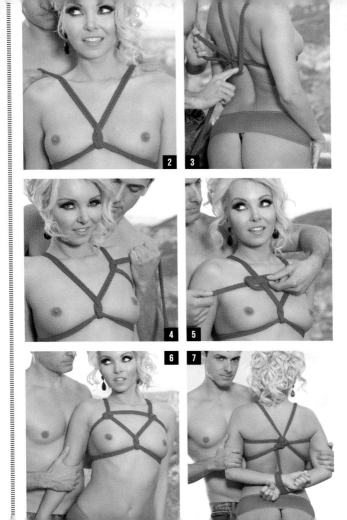

WRIST CAPTURE

This is a fun variation on the previous tie, taking it to a whole new level!

1. If you want to take the chest harness a little further, don't tie her hands behind her back. Have them relax at her sides and put another loop around them down lower, trapping the arms just above the wrists.

2. Bring the rope around through the rope running down the middle of her back, then come back the way you came.

3. Come back to the wrist and feed the rope on the inside of the wrist.

4. Bring it up and around and back through the way you just came, cinching the wrists snugly. Then go back around and do the other wrist.

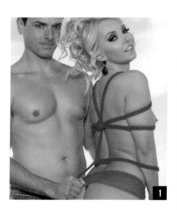

5. Come back around the rope, down the spine, and make a loop around it.

6. Knot it all off in the back and make it nice and neat.

7. She's now snug and secure and ready for a spanking!

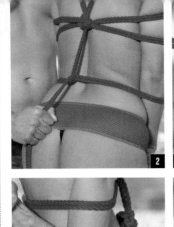

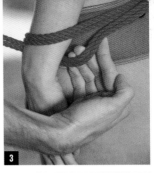

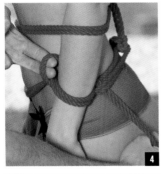

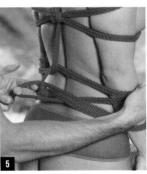

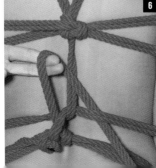

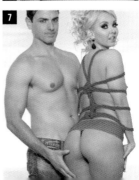

NOVICE CHEST HARNESS

Here's a chest harness that is the next step up in complexity but still easy enough to make sexy. It is a great way to gain control over your sub's upper body.

1. Start with a Lark's Head knot (page 56) around her rib cage.

2. Wrap twice around the ribs right below the breasts.

3. Make two wraps above the breasts.

4. Pull the free end through the loops you made earlier.

5. Go over the shoulder and down between the breasts, picking up the lower wraps, and then give an extra twist as you come back up over the right shoulder.

6. When you come to the back, you can tie it off and take the leftover rope to weave it back and forth up the shoulder ropes

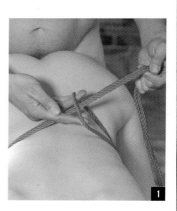

you just made. It looks neat and sexy this way.

7. Now that her top half is bound in your rope, use it as a harness to grab on to and have your way with her!

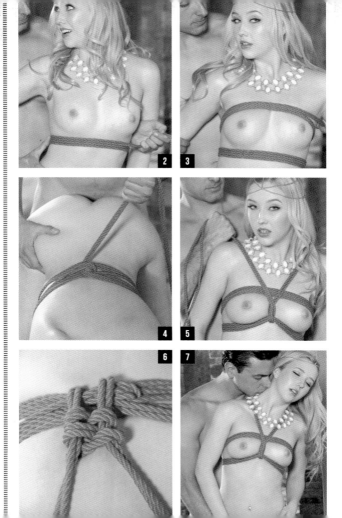

HIP HARNESS AND LEG WEAVE

This tie is more complex but not too hard. Plus it doubles as a sex harness.

1. Start with a Lark's Head knot (page 56) around the waist.

2. Wrap it around the waist twice and make a half hitch on the hip.

3. Bring the rope across the front of her thigh, down between her legs, and up in the crease of her bum, all the way up to the original hitch. Go over the wrap you just made and **under** the waist wraps and then **over** the next part of the waist and then **under** the last one.

4. Repeat, following the same path, making the opposite weave right beside the line you are following.

5. You can use another length of rope and wind down and

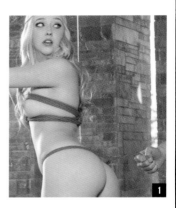

around the thigh and leg. Remember to weave opposite as you trace back through.

6. All these ropes make for great grab points during sex.

7. Use this tie to pull your partner in close and keep her there!

2

3

4

5

6

7

NOVICE SEX HARNESS HIP TIE

Want more control during sex? This hip harness provides multiple leverage points to get your partner exactly where you want him or her. The weaving technique makes it comfortable and the knots minimal.

1. Start with a simple hip wrap twice around the body and finish with a Bula Bula (page 54) or a Sommerville Bowline (page 60) in the front.

2. Come over the thigh, under the bum, and up between the legs.

3. Meet that thigh rope with a quick and easy Munter Hitch (page 58) and pull through.

4. Bring that rope around the back and make a quick hitch to keep the rope above the ass.

5. Pull it around to the front, down between the legs, up over the ass, and meet that first rope with another Munter Hitch.

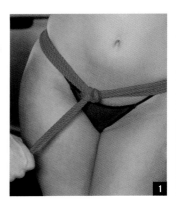

6. Take the free end and pull it up into the knot in the middle of the waist wrap; cross over and up.

7. Pull on those ropes for better leverage while thrusting.

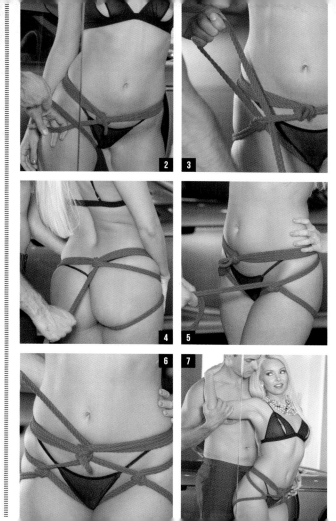

THE INFINITY

Now that you have something to grab on to, let's create another tie that uses simple weaving to accentuate the breasts.

1. Put a wrap around the chest, coming up and over one breast.

2. Change direction. Come around the front and go up and over the other breast.

3. Repeat, building on the last. Weave in and out as you cross over each new wrap.

4. Keep the back nice and neat, and when you have about 3 feet (0.91 m) left of rope, split the pair in your hand and come up and over the shoulders to the front.

5. Weave the rope down into the top wraps. This will keep it from falling.

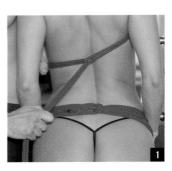

6. Try to keep it neat when you come back to the original knot. You can even use a bow to finish the tie.

7. Time to admire your partner— and your own handiwork.

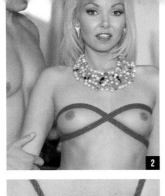
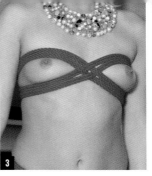
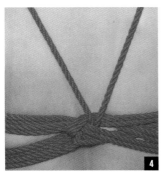
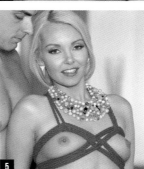
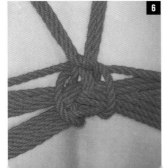
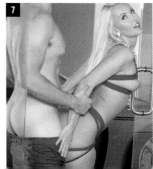

SEXY BODY TIE OR KARADA

This tie uses a series of knots to form attractive diamond patterns across the body, known as a *Karada*. It is a great way to decorate and make your partner feel attractive.

1. Start with anoverhand knot about a foot (30.5 cm) down in the rope at the bight end.

2. Slip it over your partner's head so the knot you just made sits on the back of the neck. Create a new knot between the collarbone and nipples.

3. Make a series of knots about 6 inches (15 cm) apart all the way down as you bring the rope between the legs and up the back, pulling the ends through the first loop.

4. With doubled-over rope, come under the arms and pull the rope through the vertical rope between each knot and then go back the way you came, opening up the diamond.

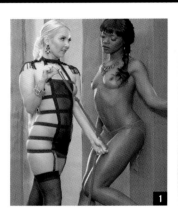

5. Wrap it around the back and come back to make the next diamond.

6. Continue down the body.

7. Your bunny is now a walking work of art.

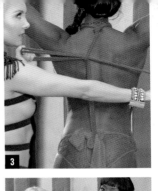

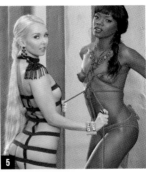

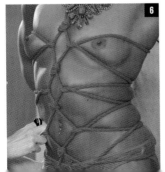

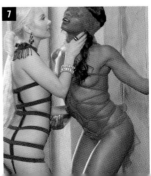

ASS OPENER

This tie for the bottom half of a woman is perfect for anal and vibrator stimulation.

1. Start with a few wraps around the body, ending in the front.

2. Make a nice simple knot around the whole series of wraps and tighten it.

3. Make two knots down the rope as it hangs in front of the pussy. The lower knot should hang in front of the clit or just below it.

4. Pull the rope up and through the waist wraps and make a knot. When you pull the ends, the back opens up. To ease into anal sex, it takes just another step or two.

5. First come around the front with each end and pull through the doubled rope across the pussy to tug the lips open.

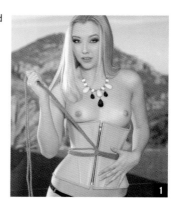

6. Pass the ropes around the back and split apart the back part of the rope, tying it off in the front around the waist.

7. Who says you can't have a hands-free orgasm?

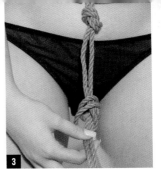

2

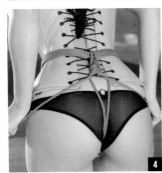

3

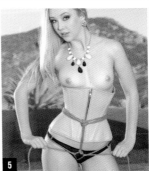

4

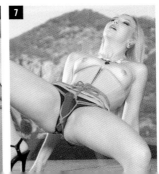

5

6

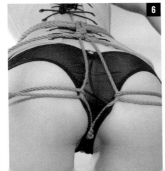

7

REDNECK TRUCKER'S HITCH

Rope your little filly into a classic spread-eagle tie to the bed. This technique uses a special hitch that you can quickly retighten at any time.

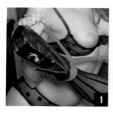 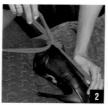 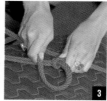

1. Start with a Bula Bula (page 54) around the ankle.

2. Make a slipknot just below the toe of the foot and go around a bedpost.

3. Come around the bedpost with the free end, feed it through the loop you just made, and pull the leg snug.

4. Pinch the first loop to hold it in place. Pull a 12-inch (30.5 cm) loop through.

5. Snug it all up.

6. You can quickly pull the loose end of to free your partner—or retighten.

7. Do this to her arms and legs.

8. This tie is just as comfortable with legs up in the air, attached to the headboard posts.

9. Here is the same tie attached to the thighs. There are a lot of positions possible with this simple technique.

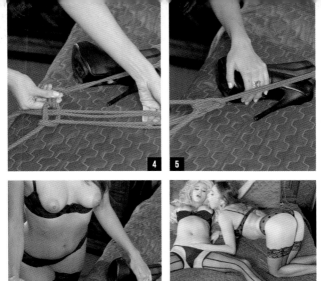

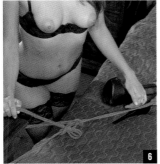

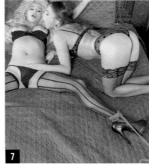

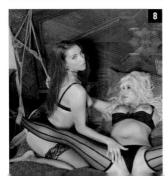

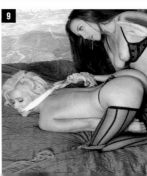

ROPE CORSET

Rope isn't just used to bind breasts in a chest tie. You can make a whole corset with enough rope. This tie is very straightforward: Once you get the first few wraps, the rest is easily repeated.

1. Start by capturing a loop around the back and pulling it to the front, keeping it above the breasts.

2. Feed the loose end through the loop and take a moment to admire your woman.

3. Bring the rope straight down between the breasts and hold it there while you come around the back to the front again.

4. Pass the loose end through the vertical rope and come right around the back again, making a full wrap.

5. Now come through the loop in the front, reverse the way you came, and . . .

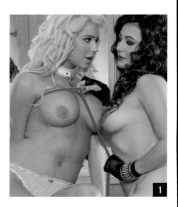

6. . . . build it all the way down by simply repeating the same pattern over and over.

7. Now your girl is pretty enough to nibble on!

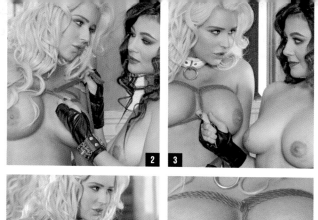

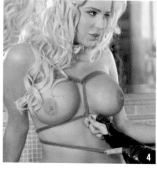

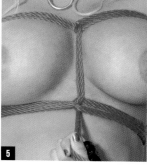

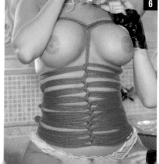

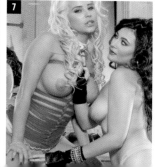

RESOURCES

Photography: Holly Randall, hollyrandall.com; Lord Morpheous, lordmorpheous.com; Geoff George Photography

Styling: Mia and AJ from Apt 9 Productions. www.apt9productions.com

Clothing: The Stockroom, 2809 ½ W. Sunset Blvd., Los Angeles, CA 90026. www.thestockroom.com; Syren Latex Fashion, www.syren.com; Stormy Leather, www.stormyleather.com

Models: Allura, Aaliyah Love, Samantha Rone, Kourtney Kane, Ryan Driller, Celeste Star, Ana Foxx, Spencer Scott, Sophia Jade, Princess, Josie, Marie McCray, Stevie Shae, Alex Chance, Zoey Monroe, Dani Daniels, and Selma Sins

Riggers: Allura, Ruairidh, and Ve-ra

ABOUT THE AUTHOR

Morpheous is a New York-based sex educator, author, photographer, and kinkster. He is the author of the popular BDSM titles *Bondage Basics, How to Be Kinky: A Beginner's Guide to BDSM, How to Be Kinkier: More Adventures in Adult Playtime*, and *How to Be Knotty: The Essential Guide to Modern Rope Bondage*. Morpheous' work is archived in the Sexual Representation Collection of the University of Toronto's Mark S. Bonham Centre for Sexual Diversity Studies, Leather Archives and Museum in Chicago, and National Archives of Canada. He is also the founder of Morpheous' Bondage Extravaganza, the world's largest public rope bondage event. You can find out more at lordmorpheous.com.